DEDICATION

I dedicate this book to everyone who has struggles in following a strict healthy diet plan. This book is a perfect guide for you on how easy it is to bring back the zest in your life.

TABLE OF CONTENTS

Healthy Lifestyle Diet with Wellness and Dietary Guide

Tips to Eat Well to a Lifestyle Diet Makeover

By: Helen Williams

9781634286862

PUBLISHERS NOTES

Disclaimer – Speedy Publishing LLC

This publication is intended to provide helpful and informative material. It is not intended to diagnose, treat, cure, or prevent any health problem or condition, nor is intended to replace the advice of a physician. No action should be taken solely on the contents of this book. Always consult your physician or qualified health-care professional on any matters regarding your health and before adopting any suggestions in this book or drawing inferences from it.

The author and publisher specifically disclaim all responsibility for any liability, loss or risk, personal or otherwise, which is incurred as a consequence, directly or indirectly, from the use or application of any contents of this book.

Any and all product names referenced within this book are the trademarks of their respective owners. None of these owners have sponsored, authorized, endorsed, or approved this book.

Always read all information provided by the manufacturers' product labels before using their products. The author and publisher are not responsible for claims made by manufacturers.

This book was originally printed before 2014. This is an adapted reprint by Speedy Publishing LLC with newly updated content designed to help readers with much more accurate and timely information and data.

Speedy Publishing LLC

40 E Main Street, Newark, Delaware, 19711

Contact Us: 1-888-248-4521

Website: http://www.speedypublishing.co

REPRINTED Paperback Edition: ISBN: 9781634286862

Manufactured in the United States of America

Chapter 1- Healthy Nutrition Plan Diet

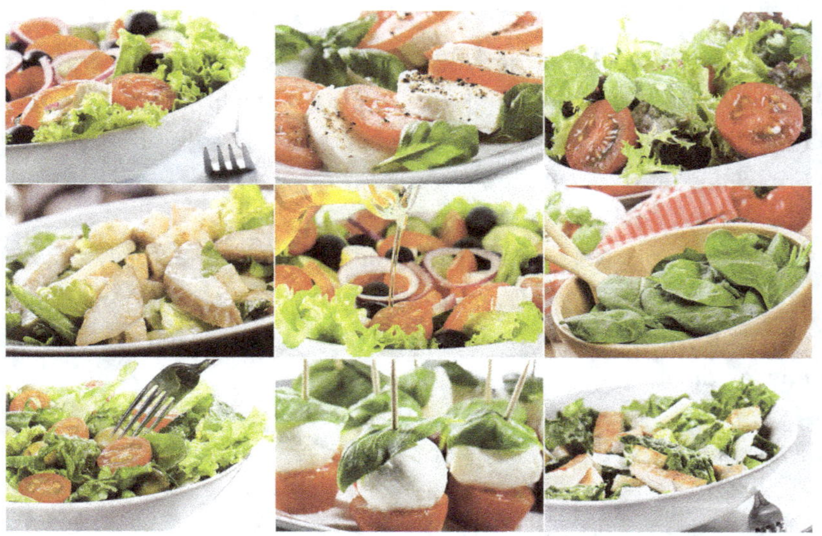

People struggle with losing weight. Sure, there are tons of reasons for this — convenience of unhealthy food, peer pressure, lack of focus, lack of dedication, lack of motivation, lack of knowledge concerning proper nutrition...

The list goes on.

You likely know several people that want to lose weight right now, or that have tried in the past. Maybe they DID lose weight, but most people that DO lose weight end up gaining most (if not all) of it back within a year.

Marketers and the media capitalize on this niche of consumers like vultures. They hawk their latest and great diet fads, contraptions for losing weight and getting in shape with increasingly less work and effort, and worst of all: everything sounds like the next best thing. (Yeah... if only.)

With new diet and weight loss books, programs, courses, and "silver-bullet" solutions coming out every single day promising rapid results with less effort than ever, where do you even start?

Well, what if I told you that you DON'T need the latest and greatest fad or contraption? What if I told you that I can break down in just these pages exactly how to lose weight – and keep it off – without breaking your back OR the bank?

One guy – Tom Ness – lost 15 pounds in 30 days (actually, it was only 28 days) using this information. In fact, it was one of the easiest things he's ever done. And now I'm going to tell you exactly how he did it.

To be blunt, you only need to do three things:

1) Restructure your diet

2) Workout in a way that burns fat while adding muscle

3) Build in a system of accountability

If you do these three things, you can't fail. In the following pages I'm going to show you the easiest ways to do all three.

First things first: if you want to lose weight, you need to immediately change how you eat.

If you're not thin and lean (or at least where you want to be), then you must realize that what or how you're currently eating is keeping you fat.

I can already hear the excuses:

"I don't eat that bad..."

"I don't want to give up some of the things I eat..."

"I don't have money to eat healthy..."

Awesome. Any more excuses? May as well get them out right now before we go on, because things need to change if you want to see results.

This isn't a "diet". "Diets" don't work because we (as a society) associate them with holding back, starvation, and pain. Even the word "diet" conjures up a mental image of a half-empty plate, hunger pains, and a set period of deprivation.

Does this sound familiar?

You see or read about a new program to get in shape and lose the pounds, so you decide to give it a go. You get all hyped up to start your new program, get everything all ready and prepare your meals in advance, and do really good for a couple days. Maybe you even make it a week. Hell, some people even make it two.

But then, one day, you wake up for work late. You didn't prepare your meal in advance and don't have time to pack anything before you leave. At work on your break, your only option is fast food because you don't have time for anything else. Either that or you're really hungry and just want something fast, so you cave for that one meal (or two).

But that night, realizing you've already blown your "diet" for the day, you decide to just make it a cheat day and splurge. Now it's

Thursday night and you've blown your nutrition out of the water. Mentally lashing yourself, you decide to renew your healthy vigor tomorrow.

But that next night – Friday night – you're invited to go out. Everyone's having a couple drinks and you obviously don't want to be the one person out NOT drinking, so you have a drink. One turns into two or three (or more), and after the bar everyone including you is hungry so you get something to eat. The only places open late are the greasy, fried places, but you've been drinking and are hungry so you say "Oh what the hell" and get something anyway.

Realizing your diet is now shot, you decide to just take the weekend off and start again on Monday. Monday will be the day; you'll do really well on Monday...

That's what happens to most people when they go on "diets". They almost set them themselves up for failure before they even begin.

Instead of "going on a diet", you need to restructure your lifestyle. Lifestyle changes last longer than diet plans because they fundamentally change what you eat and how you view your health and nutrition.

Sure, you can go on a "diet plan" for let's say 30 days and follow it to the letter. But what happens after those 30 days (if you even make it there)? Are you just going to do that plan again, and again?

After you stop, unless you've changed your habits – your lifestyle – you're going to revert to your older, unhealthy habits that you've spent the last 30 days trying to undo.

That's why you need to develop the mentality that this is a lifestyle change. You need a permanent solution to nutrition, which comes down to proper education and a game plan to be healthy.

You don't want a limited-time solution; you need a permanent one that will allow you to get the pounds off and keep them off, and NOT gain everything back as soon as you finish the program.

With all of that said, let me tell you exactly how Tom personally restructured his diet to drop pounds almost effortlessly – while still feeling full most of the time!

The 5 Pillars of Losing Weight

Here are the basics of this program. Consider these the "Pillars" of this reconstruction phase:

Pillar #1: Stick to five 400-calorie meals per day.

Here's an unpopular fact: there's a strong correlation between the calories you consume and how much you weight. (Crazy, eh?)

However, this is the most important part of this program since it's what you actually consume on a daily basis. If you're going to lose weight, you need to regulate what you eat. You need to know what's being consumed and what it's doing for your body.

For the first week of this program, eat four 400-calorie meals and drink at least 8 cups of water each day (I'd recommend drinking even more than that). This is to reduce the amount of food traveling in your body and "clean" you out. Consider this your healthy body cleanse.

After the first week, eat five 400-calorie meals. Note that you're consuming the same amount of calories each meal, you're just eating one more meal each day than you were in the first week.

Not only does this breakdown make for a consistent meal plan, it also makes each meal that much more important. If you only have 1,600-2,000 calories to work with each day, you need to make sure you're planning them out correctly so your body gets the proper nutrition.

Pillar #2: Make sure you consume Monounsaturated Fats with every meal.

Not all fats are created equal. Yes, you want to avoid some fats like Trans Fat. To scare yourself, go ahead and Google "why is trans fat bad?" I'll leave that one to Google to tell you.

So what about good fat? Those would be the monounsaturated fats.

You'll find monounsaturated fats most prevalently in these foods:

• Oils (olive oil, almond oil, sesame oil, flax oil, etc)

• Avocados

• Olives

• Nuts and seeds (almonds, walnuts, sunflower seeds, etc)

• Dark Chocolate (yes, this is everyone's favorite among these)

Monounsaturated fats have a whole slew of healthy benefits, but one of the most attractive ones is that they help promote fat loss.

Best of all, you can easily incorporate one of these foods into every meal you eat. In fact, you need to for this program.

Pillar #3: Eat slowly.

Fact: when you slam your food, it doesn't last as long nor is it as filling as it could be. Eating fast doesn't curb hunger as well as eating the same portion slowly, which can lead to over-eating or feeling unfulfilled, resulting in over-eating later.

Instead of rushing to be the first one done with your plate, take your time. Eat your food slowly and you'll feel more satisfied with the same amount of food (as opposed to eating it faster and not feeling satisfied).

Also, drink a full glass of water before each meal and if possible drink another full glass during or after you finish your meal. This will help you feel fuller without over-eating.

Pillar #4: Drink lots of water.

This should be a staple of your day-to-day lifestyle anyway, so it should go without saying that water needs to be the main liquid you consume.

Not only is water essential to a healthy body and hydration, but it can help fill you up (odd as that sounds). I mentioned this in the last point above, but when you drink water before, during or after your meals, it helps satisfy hunger cravings.

In addition, drinking water periodically helps curb your appetite throughout the day, making it easier to stick to a balanced diet with proper nutrition.

Case in point: drink more water!

Pillar #5: Prepare meals in advance.

Most people don't fall off the healthy band wagon because they want to, but because they plan poorly (or don't plan at all).

Remember the age-old saying: "Fail to plan, plan to fail". The anonymous creator of that saying couldn't have been more right.

To be successful on any meal plan – dietary or otherwise – you need to prepare foods and/or in advance. When I know I'm working in the morning, there is a very slim chance I'll allow time to pack a proper meal plan to eat throughout the day before I leave, so I make sure to do it before I go to bed. That way, I just get up and grab the bag out of the refrigerator and I'm good to go.

Chapter 2- Always Go for Healthy Food for Healthy Lifestyle

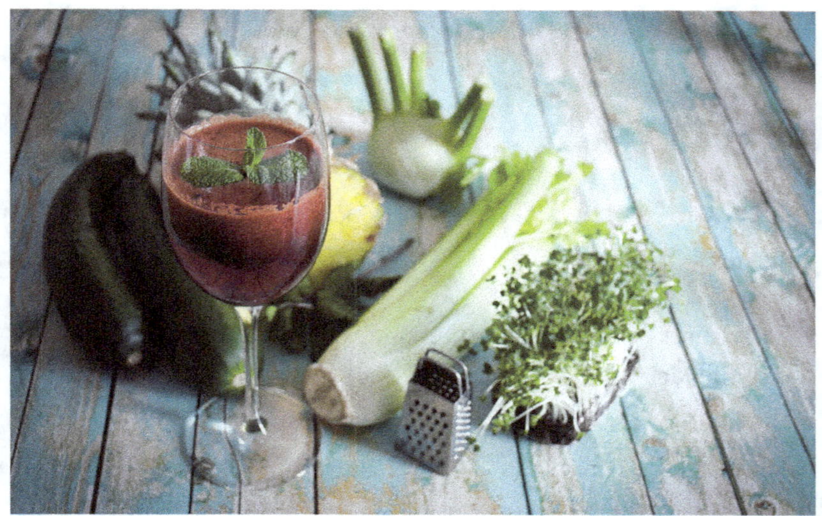

There are certain foods you should eat on this plan. They're designed to be healthy and pack in all the nutrients you need (or close enough), and they can be very filling as well.

- The List Itself -

• Ground turkey (or ground chicken)

• Lean Ground Beef

• Non-fat Greek yogurt (I prefer Oikos Greek Nonfat Vanilla Yogurt)

• Other non-fat dairy

• Raw Nuts / Seeds (almonds, walnuts, cashews, sunflower seeds, etc)

• Eggs

- Apples

- Bananas

- Sweet Potatoes (and other orange vegetables like carrots)

- Salsa

- Avocados

- Berries

- All-Natural peanut butter (the kind with the oil separated at the top of the jar)

- Corn Tortillas

- Beans and Lentils

- Dark Chocolate

- Broccoli (and other cruciferous vegetables)

- Mushrooms

- Black coffee and tea

- Tomatoes

- Salmon (and other fish higher in Omega 3)

- Flank Steak (or Top Round)

- Plain oatmeal

You're not limited to just these foods, but there are five general rules you'll want to follow beyond the list above.

5 Very Important Rules Beyond "The List":

1) Make generally healthier choices

2) Eat more natural, unprocessed foods

3) Minimize the sodium you consume

4) Reduce the amount of carbs you consume

5) Keep your meals around 400 calories

These are general guidelines, but you'll need to stick to them fairly closely if you want to see lasting results.

Again, from the "Pillars" above, make sure that you incorporate a monounsaturated fat with every meal.

How To Sneak a Monounsaturated Fat In Any Meal:

• drizzling olive oil over a salad (instead of regular dressing)

• cooking your foods in oil

• adding a serving of nuts, seeds, or dark chocolate into yogurt

• Slicing up half an avocado and putting the slices on a sandwich

• Make a breakfast sandwich with eggs, a whole wheat English muffin, and a few avocado slices (you can even add 1-2 tablespoons of salsa to add flavor)

I'm sure you can get more creative, but that's just what I typically do and it works out really well.

Better yet: mash up the avocados, add a sprinkle of garlic powder, half a fresh, diced tomato, as much cilantro as you can handle, and a dash of lime juice. This is the recipe for some amazing guacamole, so add it to anything you make to make it instantly amazing.

Time and Eat Right

There's going to come a time when you have to rush out the door and don't have time to make breakfast or lunch. What if you need something on the go?

You can't just go without eating, so it's wise to plan for the situations where you need to grab something and go. Contrary to what a lot of people think, this doesn't have to mean fast food; in fact, there are some delicious alternatives that you can throw in a bag to satisfy hunger or even just supplement a small snack if you can't wait till lunch or dinner.

Protein bars are a great way to pack nutrition in something you can grab out of a cabinet in a hurry. You could also put a couple scoops of high-quality protein powder into a zip-lock bag to make a shake for a snack. Simply pour the powder in a medium-sized cup of water and stir it up.

• Healthy (and good-tasting) Protein Bars – QUEST Bar (apple pie is my favorite flavor)

• Meal Replacement Shakes (Protein Powder) – SPECIES Isolyze or OPTIMUM NUTRITION Platinum HydroWhey (mix 1-2 scoops in water or milk)

• The Best "Any time" Snack – BelVita Breakfast biscuits (Blueberry is crazy good)

Chapter 3- Healthy Lifestyle, Diet and Wellness

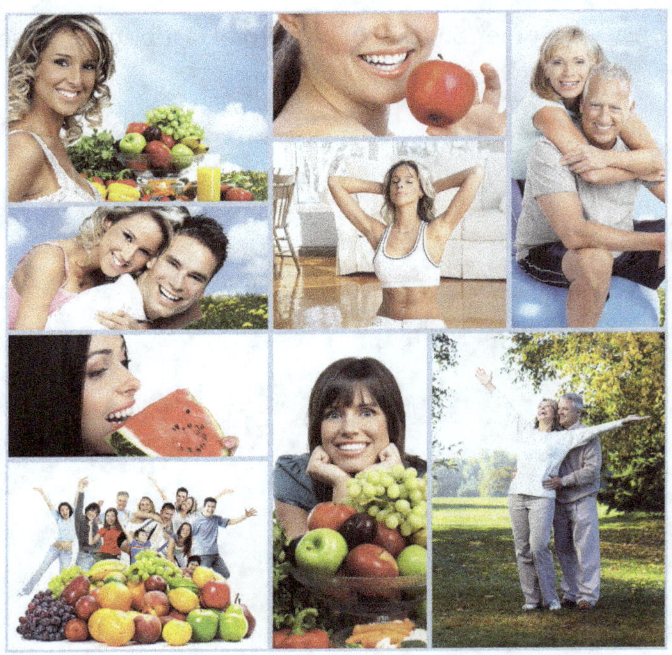

The one main thing to remember about supplements is that they aren't necessary, but in some cases they can help speed things up or "fill in the gaps" in your nutrition. This really depends on what you're trying to accomplish and what you're doing to accomplish it.

- Protein -

For example, if you work out a lot or lift weights, then you may want to take a protein supplement (a shake or protein bar) after working out. You generally want to consume protein within 30 minutes of every workout. Here's an excellent powder to take for this:

• High-Quality Protein Powder – SPECIES Isolyze or OPTIMUM NUTRITION Platinum HydroWhey (same one from Chapter 4 above)

However, if you don't incorporate working out in your schedule, then you'll likely get all the protein you need from the foods I mentioned on the list in Chapter 3. Just make sure to incorporate a lean protein with every meal. You don't benefit from an excess of protein, and studies have shown that it can even keep the weight on.

- Probiotics / Digestive Enzymes -

I recommend taking probiotics daily along with digestive enzymes at every meal to make sure your body is breaking down and fully absorbing each meal. You can see much better results this way.

• Probiotics – JARROW Jarro-Dophilus EPS

• Digestive Enzymes – NOW Super Enzymes

- Fish Oil -

If you do not like eating fish, I recommend getting a good quality fish oil supplement that comes in the form of capsules.

• Fish Oil – OPTIMUM NUTRITION Fish Oil

- Creatine -

You'll hear this supplement mentioned all the time, but few people know what it really is for. If you're looking to pack on muscle and excel muscle growth to bulk up, you'll want to take this.

However, if you don't have a low enough body fat to make out muscle density – or if you're just looking to drop weight and lean out – then creatine won't benefit you in any significant way.

Because of this, I'd only recommend taking it when you're lean and want to add muscle.

One of the best times to take creatine is when you ARE lean with lower body fat and crank up the intensity of your weight lifting. The muscles grow at more rapid rate on this supplement, so used in conjunction with a workout where you focus on heavy weight and low reps; you will achieve an extremely ripped physique in a short amount of time.

(Hint: This would be a perfect plan 1-2 months before beach season, wouldn't it?)

The Secret Sauce

If diet programs are so great, why do even the die-hard dieters often fall off the bandwagon and drop the dietary ball?

The reason is accountability.

Accountability is the "secret sauce" for this program. It's what keeps you motivated, focused and on track. It makes you conscious of what you're eating, guilty when you're cheating, and eager to get back on track.

Here are the exact steps to take to ensure you stay accountable on this program:

Accountability Step #1: Tell everyone what you're doing.

When you set your mind to doing something and you're the only one that knows about it, it's easy to back out of following through and committing to it.

But when you commit to doing something and your entire family and friend base know about it, you'll find it's a little harder to back out of it.

That's why it's critical that when you actually decide to losing weight and start a program like this, you NEED to set up built-in mechanisms that keep you going. Fortunately, it's as easy as telling everyone what you're going to do.

If you're going to lose 15 pounds in 30 days (or whatever it is you're going to do), tell everyone. Make it known. That way, when you feel like quitting – which you may quite possibly feel at one point or another – you're not just quitting on yourself; you're quitting on everyone you told about your commitment.

Accountability Step #2: Take your starting measurements AND PICTURES.

This is a BIG one, and one I have ignored in the past. When you first start a program, you need to know where you are with your weight and measurements. This "system check" is extremely important because otherwise as you progress through the program you won't know how you're improving.

It's like making sure there's gas in your car before you start a road trip. Would you just start driving, or check to make sure you have a full tank? (You'd obviously check to make sure you have a full tank, and any diet program is no different.)

You'll also want to take pictures in addition to measurements. You've seen these before: they're the "Before & After" pictures from people before they started the program and then after they've finished it. You'll likely want to skip this step, but you can't afford to. Those "before" pictures are meant to be a visual accountability check. Put them in a highly visible place - like on your bathroom mirror - somewhere you'll see them every day.

You want to be reminded of your physical condition every day as it will motivate you to improve it. Then, as you progress through the program and take "update" pictures, you'll see your improvement and you'll be motivated to continue the program.

Here are the poses to take for these pictures:

a) Facing front (arms down, abs un-flexed)

b) Facing front (arms up, biceps flexed)

c) Facing the side (arms down, abs un-flexed)

d) Facing the back (arms up, biceps flexed)

Take pictures in these poses before you start the program, once or twice throughout your program, and after you complete it (after the 30 days). You'll see the improvements - and know exactly how you got there, since you've been tracking everything the last 30 days.

Accountability Step #3: Track everything you eat on a daily basis.

Remember that saying, "What doesn't get measured doesn't get improved?" Yeah, well, there's more truth to that than you realize.

Measuring your progress is the cornerstone for improvement. If you keep track of what you eat, you're likewise accountable for what you eat. This way, you can't be surprised when you gain or lose weight since you can see exactly what you had that caused the fluctuation. If you gained weight, you'll know why. If you lost weight, you'll know why for that too.

It would be extremely tedious if you had to manually write down every single thing you ate all day, and then go in and fill in all the nutrition contents of those foods.

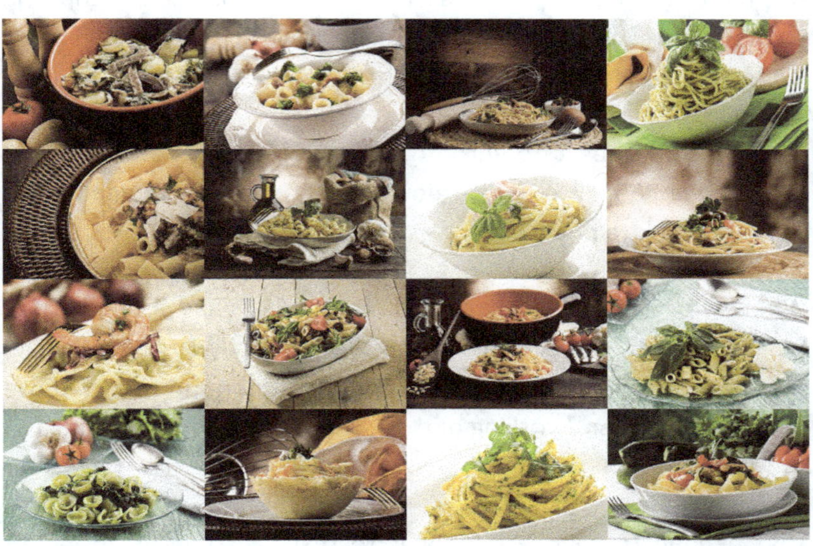

What are you working towards? Why are you losing weight? And more importantly: why do you need to do it NOW instead of later?

These are all extremely important questions. The main catalyst behind Tom's weight loss was that he was going on a trip and wanted to look good for it. (Well really, it was for a special lady he was going to be seeing when he got there.)

Tom had four weeks to get into shape, and knew he didn't have time to kill; he had to hunker down and do what he needed to do to drop the extra pounds.

What helped more than anything was that he had a deadline of four weeks to do this. Tom has said that he's always been active, but he's never had the best dietary habits. Even I'm one of those people that's been "working out" for years, but don't have much to show for it.

That needed to change if he was to reach his goal of losing 15 pounds in only four weeks. Using the exact strategies laid out in this program, he was able to drop those pounds and keep them off.

CHAPTER 4- PLAN AND WORKOUT PLAN FOR YOUR WELLNESS

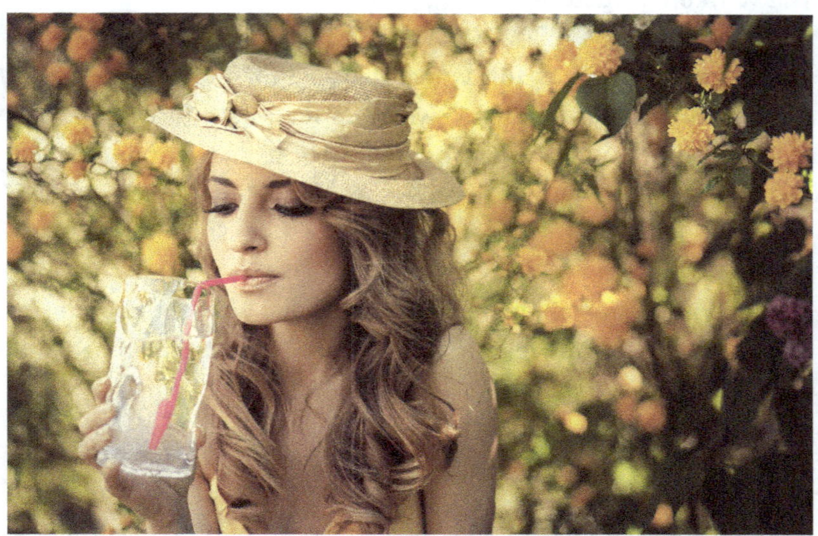

The Non-Cardio Cardio Workout That Shreds Body Fat

If you stick to the meal plan alone, you can see results. In fact, that's how Tom lost most of the 15 pounds in only 30 days.

But if you want to really ramp things up and burn more body fat, you'll want to introduce working out into your schedule.

If you want to maximize fat loss without spending hours in the gym (or on a treadmill), the solution for you is circuit training. Circuit training is a cardio-style workout where you do 1-2 series of several exercises back-to-back with no rest in between the sets or exercises.

When you lift like this, the workout itself becomes more aerobic and cardiovascular, burning more calories without actually doing "cardio" - like running or jogging.

Aim to work out 4 days a week if you're going to introduce working out into your schedule.

The Workout Structure

There are two parts to this workout. You'll follow one routine for the first two weeks and then switch up for weeks three and four. This will prevent your body from adjusting to the routine and will make the exercises more effective, especially in conjunction with the Diet program.

This is how I'd recommend structuring your workout routine for maximum effect (this workout was designed by a certified personal trainer, by the way):

Weeks 1 & 2

• Monday: Chest / Triceps (+ Abs)

• Wednesday: Back / Biceps (+ Abs)

• Friday: Shoulders (+ Abs)

• Saturday: Legs

...And to break down each day's exercises:

Monday:

Chest / Triceps Circuit Exercises

Instructions: For each muscle group, perform one set of 8-10 reps for all the exercises straight through with no rest between exercises. That's one "series". Rest 1-2 minutes after completing a full series, then repeat it (for a total of two series).

You should be using weights heavy enough that 8-10 reps bring you to failure for the given exercises. If you can't get up at least in the 6-8 range, you're going too heavy, and if you can get up more than 10 reps easily then you're going too light.

As you progress through the series, you'll likely have to drop the weight you're using to hit the appropriate rep range as muscle fatigue will set in.

- Chest -

• Incline dumbbell press

• Flat dumbbell press

• decline dumbbell press

• Incline dumbbell fly

• Flat dumbbell fly

• Cable crossovers

- Triceps -

• Rope Push Downs

• Straight Bar (or V-Bar) Pushdowns

• Skull Crushers

• 2-Arm Overhead Dumbbell Extensions (seated)

• Unilateral Push Downs (do one arm at a time)

- Abs - (Do these after the series above)

• Twisting Sit Ups – 2 x 20 reps (crossing up to each side is a rep)

• Knee Raises – 2 x 20 reps (Use a Roman Chair or hanging)

• Side Bends – 2 x 15 reps

Wednesday:

Back / Biceps Circuit Exercises

Instructions: For each muscle group, perform one set of 8-10 reps for all the exercises straight through with no rest between exercises (again, use heavy enough weights that 8-10 reps bring you to failure). That's one "series". Rest 1-2 minutes after completing a full series, then repeat it (for a total of two series).

- Back -

• Pull Downs (wide grip)

• Bent Over Barbell Rows (wide grip)

• Bent Over Barbell Rows (close grip, hands about 6-8 inches apart)

• Reverse Grip Pull Downs

• Seated Cable Rows

• Straight Arm Pull Down

- Biceps –

• Standing Barbell Curl (wide grip)

• Standing Barbell Curl Close Grip (hands spaced 8 inches apart)

• Seated Dumbbell Curl

• Incline Dumbbell Curl

• Hammer Curls

• Standing Cable Curls

- Abs - (Do these after the series above)

• Decline Sit Ups – 2 x 20 reps (Use a slant board for these)

• Weighted Knee Raises – 2 x 15 reps (Use a Roman Chair with a light dumbbell)

• Side Bends – 2 x 15 reps

Friday:

Shoulders Circuit Exercises

Instructions: For each muscle group, perform one set of 8-10 reps for all the exercises straight through with no rest between exercises (again, use heavy enough weights that 8-10 reps bring you to failure). That's one "series". Rest 1-2 minutes after completing a full series, then repeat it (for a total of two series).

- Shoulders -

• Seated Dumbbell Press

• Standing Dumbbell Lateral Raise

• Unilateral Cable Lateral Raise (one arm at a time)

• Upright Rows (close grip)

• Front Dumbbell Raise

• Shrugs (using a barbell)

- Abs - (Do these after the series above)

• Standard Crunches – 2 x 25 reps (or till failure)

• Planks – 3 x 1 minute

Saturday:

Legs Circuit Exercises

Instructions: For each muscle group, perform one set of 8-10 reps for all the exercises straight through with no rest between exercises (again, use heavy enough weights that 8-10 reps bring you to failure). That's one "series". Rest 1-2 minutes after completing a full series, then repeat it (for a total of two series).

- Quads -

• Leg Extensions

• Leg Press (feet close together)

• Leg Press (feet placed high and wide)

• Hack Squat (feet close together)

• Hack Squat (feet wide)

• Lunges (using a Smith Machine or walking)

- Hamstrings -

• Lying Leg Curl

• Seated Leg Curl

Follow this plan for the first two weeks. After that, we're going to switch it up...

Weeks 3 & 4

• Monday: Back / Biceps (+ Abs)

• Wednesday: Legs

• Friday: Chest / Triceps (+ Abs)

• Saturday: Shoulders (+ Abs)

Here's how these workouts look like:

Monday:

Back / Biceps Circuit Exercises

Instructions: For each muscle group, perform one set of 8-10 reps for all the exercises straight through with no rest between exercises (again, use heavy enough weights that 8-10 reps bring you to failure). That's one "series". Rest 1-2 minutes after completing a full series, then repeat it (for a total of two series).

- Back -

• Pull Downs (wide grip)

• Reverse Grip Pull Downs

• Seated Cable Rows

• Straight Arm Pull Down

• Bent Over Barbell Rows (wide grip)

• Bent Over Barbell Rows (close grip, hands about 6-8 inches apart)

- Biceps –

• Seated Dumbbell Curl

• Incline Dumbbell Curl

• Hammer Curls

• Standing Barbell Curl (wide grip)

• Standing Barbell Curl Close Grip (hands spaced 8 inches apart)

• Standing Cable Curls

- Abs - (Do these after the series above)

• Decline Sit Ups – 2 x 20 reps (Use a slant board for these)

• Weighted Knee Raises – 2 x 15 reps (Use a Roman Chair with a light dumbbell)

• Side Bends – 2 x 15 reps

Wednesday:

Legs Circuit Exercises

Instructions: For each muscle group, perform one set of 8-10 reps for all the exercises straight through with no rest between exercises (again, use heavy enough weights that 8-10 reps bring you to failure). That's one "series". Rest 1-2 minutes after completing a full series, then repeat it (for a total of two series).

- Quads -

• Leg Press (feet close together)

• Leg Press (feet placed high and wide)

• Leg Extensions

• Hack Squat (feet close together)

• Hack Squat (feet wide)

• Lunges (using a Smith Machine or walking)

- Hamstrings -

• Seated Leg Curl

• Lying Leg Curl

- Abs - (Do these after the series above)

• Standard Sit Ups – 2 x 20 reps (Use a slant board if possible)

• Side Bends – 2 x 15 reps

Friday:

Chest / Triceps Circuit Exercises

Instructions: As with Weeks 1 and 2, for each muscle group perform one set of 8-10 reps for all the exercises straight through with no rest between exercises. That's one "series". Rest 1-2 minutes after completing a full series, then repeat it (for a total of two series).

You should still be using weights heavy enough that 8-10 reps bring you to failure for the given exercises. If you can't get up at least in the 6-8 range, you're going too heavy, and if you can get up more than 10 reps easily then you're going too light.

As you progress through the series, you'll likely have to drop the weight you're using to hit the appropriate rep range as muscle fatigue will set in.

- Chest -

• Incline dumbbell fly

• flat dumbbell fly

• Cable crossovers

• Incline dumbbell press

• Flat dumbbell press

• decline dumbbell press

- Triceps -

• 2-Arm Overhead Dumbbell Extensions (seated)

• Unilateral Push Downs (do one arm at a time)

• Rope Push Downs

• Straight Bar (or V-Bar) Pushdowns

• Skull Crushers

- Abs - (Do these after the series above)

• Twisting Sit Ups – 2 x 20 reps (crossing up to each side is a rep)

• Knee Raises – 2 x 20 reps (Use a Roman Chair or hanging)

• Side Bends – 2 x 15 reps

Saturday:

Shoulders Circuit Exercises

Instructions: For each muscle group, perform one set of 8-10 reps for all the exercises straight through with no rest between exercises (again, use heavy enough weights that 8-10 reps bring you to failure). That's one "series". Rest 1-2 minutes after completing a full series, then repeat it (for a total of two series).

- Shoulders -

• Unilateral Cable Lateral Raise (one arm at a time)

• Upright Rows (close grip)

• Seated Dumbbell Press

• Standing Dumbbell Lateral Raise

• Front Dumbbell Raise

• Shrugs (using a barbell)

- Abs - (Do these after the series above)

• Standard Crunches – 2 x 25 reps (or till failure)

• Planks – 2 x 1 minute

• Side Planks – 2 x 1 minute (on each side)

This is it for the routine for Weeks 3 and 4. As you can see, it's the same exercises but they're done in a different order and on different days of the week. This will confuse your muscles which will avoid plateaus, allowing you to continue to make gains and shred body fat with this workout – even after the first couple weeks.

As you progress through this workout, increase the weights if they're getting lighter so you can hit the appropriate rep range for the given exercises. Despite the muscle fatigue you'll experience further into each of the series, you'll gain strength over the course of this program from using heavier weights.

Diet and Exercise for Immediate Result

With any workout program, there are ways to get better and faster results. Here are a couple ways to maximize this program even more:

Add Exercises To The Series

One of the easiest tactics to get more bangs for your buck is to increase the number of exercises you do in the series throughout this program (for each muscle group). There is any number of unique exercises out there that you can find by simply looking through exercise books, websites or magazines.

I wouldn't exceed 10 exercises total for the series, but this program features 6 per muscle group, so you have some room to work with.

Incorporate Cardio Into Your Workouts

Nobody likes to hear this, but it's a fact: incorporating cardio into your workouts can rapidly accelerate your fat loss and speed things up.

I'd recommend doing 30 minutes of cardio after each of your non-leg workouts (so that would mean do cardio after your shoulders, chest/triceps, and back/biceps).

Now before you form that mental image of walking endlessly on a treadmill, you need to know that there are tons of different ways you can get in 30 minutes of cardio.

For example, I love to play racquetball and I'm really good at it. It also happens to burn more calories than even running for an equivalent amount of time, but it's WAY more fun to do.

Intensity Interval Training

This is one of the most effective forms of cardio you can do in conjunction with this program. Intensity Interval Training is where you do an exercise for a set amount of time, and then kicks up the intensity to get your heart rate up, and then lower the intensity to drop it back down.

This is what I'd recommend for this program:

Start out by walking on a treadmill for 3 minutes on an incline of 3-6. Then jog for 2 minutes at a 2-3 incline. That's one "interval". Repeat this 6 more times for a total of 30 minutes.

Right there is 30 minutes of cardio, but because you're switching it up every 2-3 minutes it's not just "boring treadmill cardio". It keeps you engaged and the time flies as a result.

The benefit of this is that because you're raising and lowering your heart rate constantly, your body will burn more calories than simply jogging at a static pace. This means you'll be able to get in the same calorie burning with a shorter cardio session.

Work Out In A Fasted State

One of the best times to work out is in the morning when your body is in what's called a "fasted state". This is when you haven't consumed any calories in several hours.

Think about it: when you're sleeping, assuming you get more than 5-6 hours of sleep at night, your body is going the entire time on zero food and calories. If you train when you wake up (cardio or weight lifting) it's more beneficial to both fat burning and muscle gaining.

So as hard as it is – especially when the alarm clock is going off in the morning – instead of hitting Snooze, get up and hit the gym to maximize your workout.

Chapter 5- Eating Habit Affects Total Wellness

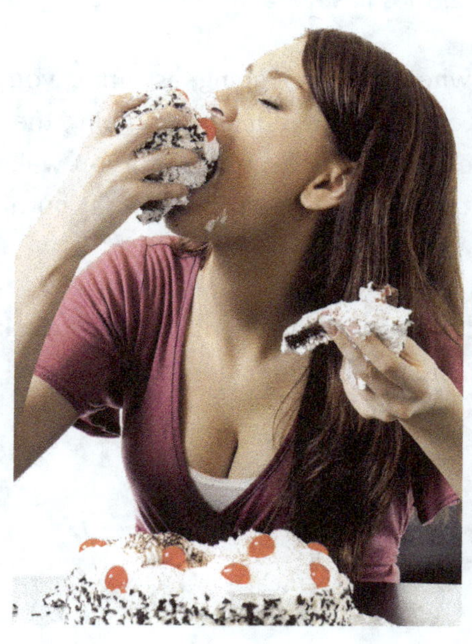

Staying healthy is a very good position to be in, as the opposite of that would be tracking in and out of hospitals with one medical condition or another. This cannot only be depressing but can also severely dent the wallet, as medical bills can be rather expensive to handle. Being able to enjoy life without the burden of popping pills and visiting doctors every so often is definitely a better option to live by.

Extensive research has shown that many medical conditions are the result of poor eating habits coupled with the lack of consistent exercise and a stress-filled life. Therefore taking the time to seriously address these issues before they turn into problems is one way of keeping healthy.

It would certainly be lighter on the wallet, when the individual is not bogged down with medical bills and the trauma of having to face a terminal condition. Poor dietary plans usually cause less that optimum body conditions, where the clogging, damaging and over working of internal body systems can then contribute to poor health conditions.

Therefore instead of having to deal with the probability of managing poor health, the better option would be to start on a healthy diet plan, a regular exercise regiment and a stress free mindset. Having some knowledge and education on the benefits of healthy living style, will not benefit the individual, if information learnt is not put into practice. As the human body naturally deteriorates as it ages all steps should be taken to ensure the process is not helped along by poor health.

Nutrition is Important

There are a lot of reasons why there are various diets available to the general public, and most of these safer diets are designed around the importance of nutrient content.

Nutrients

Nutrition is the key factor to a healthy body system which is able to function at its optimum capabilities and also help to maintain an ideal positive overall health condition. One way of ensuring the right nutrition intake is practiced, that the measured amount considered being enough for the individual is to ensure the diet plan includes elements such as carbohydrates, fats, fibers, minerals, proteins, vitamins and water. Good nutrition intake is even more beneficial to specific parts of the body and not just the overall body system.

The following are just some ways of how specific the benefits can be: The heart of course is the essential core of the entire body system; therefore being of such important is needs the special attention so that is cab function at its optimum, thus the need for good nutritional support.

The bones are basically the elements that keep everything together. Here to there is a need for good nutritional support as without optimum bone density and quality the body will experience a lot of connective problems.

Energy for the body is derived from the daily food intake, and there is a need to ensure this food is nutritionally based so that the relevant minerals and vitamins can be dispersed within the system to churn out the necessary energy source for the body's energy needs.

With good nutrition the human body can function at its optimum and basically be able to "last" and with stand any adverse effects the surroundings may throw at it. Often people disregard the importance of good nutrition and this is especially prevalent among the youngsters who seem to think their health in infallible.

What's Needed?

• Vitamin A – found in milk, cheese, cream, liver, kidney and certain types of fish oils. These have high content of saturated fats and cholesterol. Vegetable that are brighter and more vibrant in color contain higher levels of beta-carotene content.

• Vitamin D – found in cheese, butter, margarine, cream, fish, oysters and skin that are exposed to controlled doses of sunlight.

• Vitamin E – found in wheat germ, corn, nuts, seeds, olives, spinach, asparagus and other leafy vegetable and vegetable oils.

• Vitamin K – found in cabbage, cauliflower, spinach, soybeans and cereals. Some bacteria in the intestinal tracks also help to produce this vitamin.

• Thiamine also known as Vitamin B1 – found in fortifies breads, cereals, pasta, whole grains, lean meats, fish, dried beans, peas and soybeans, dairy products, certain fruits and vegetables.

• Niacin also known as Vitamin B3 – found in dairy products, poultry, fish, lean meats, nuts, legumes and enriched breads and cereals.

• Folate – found in green, leafy vegetables and many foods which are now fortified with this.

• Vitamin B12 – found in eggs, meats, poultry, shellfish and milk or milk based products.

• Pantothenic acid and biotin – found in eggs, fish, dairy products, whole grain cereals, legumes, yeast, broccoli and other vegetables in the cabbage family, white and sweet potatoes, lean beef and other similar category foods.

Chapter 6- Food Choices Depicts your Lifestyle

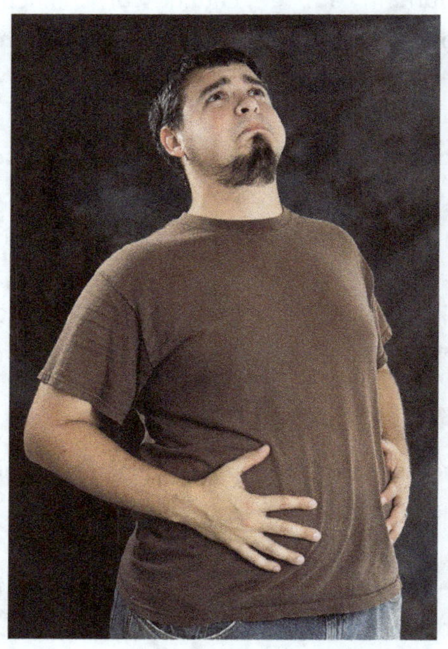

Everyone has a different take on the good and bad attributes of having a diet plan low in calorie count. However it would be better for the individual to explore the best calorie plan that is suited for his or her own lifestyle rather that to adopt just any calorie plan in the hope of staying at an optimally healthy level.

Have A Look

Calories are not bad for the body, in fact they are a necessity as they function as the provider of the energy source for the daily body's needs. The problem lies in the actual intake of calories, where the intake is more than the usage of energy, thus contributing to a high percentage of the unused calorie being stored in the body system and this then contributes to the negative side effects which cause weight gain.

All foods contain calories the only difference is some of these food contain higher amounts of calories than others. The usual measurement of the calorie content would be 1 gram of calorie is broken down into these following contributing measurements – carbohydrate is 4 calories, protein is 4 calories and fat is 9 calories.

Most food product sold will carry the above breakdown for the shopper to have an idea of the calorie content of the item being bought for consumption purposes. Therefore in the quest to watch the calories it would be product to start taking note of the information divulged on the packaging.

A fairly good guideline to go by would be that most green have comparably lower calories content to other foods. Often the sweetened or processed foods have very high calorie content and this is also only slightly less when it comes to the calorie content in meats.

The fattier the meats the higher the calorie content therefore it would be better to opt for as much lean meat intake as possible.

Most children and youngsters don't really need to watch their calorie intake if they practice very active daily routines but for the working adult without any or much physical workouts in the routine watching calories would be something to seriously consider.

Live A Healthy Lifestyle

There are a lot of opinions on how to live a healthy lifestyle, for some it would mean eating only certain foods and following a strict diet plan, for others it would mean a lot of physical exercise and yet for others it would mean living a stress free lifestyle.

All these have its good attributes and are really quite advantages to follow but none can create a healthy lifestyle scenario by itself, ideally it should be a combination of all different positive elements complimenting each other to create the healthy lifestyle.

Getting Started

Taking small steps is often a better way to start the healthy lifestyle journey as it does entail some very significant changes. For most people who have go at it all at once, the fee ing of being overwhelmed and defeated often causes them to eventually abandon any attempt to pursue a healthy lifestyle reg ment.

Making simple adjustments without any drastic eliminating exercises will help to encourage the individual to make further more significant changes as time goes on. These simple steps may include adding more greens and fruits to the current dietary habits.

Cutting down on unhealthy processed snacks is a good step to initiate but is often very difficult as these foods are usually delicious and hard to resist as they are so fittingly named "comfort foods", however one way to doing so successfully is not having such food readily available and within easy reach. The next time the grocery shopping is done, making an effort not to add these items to the cart would be a good first step in the right direction.

Another small change that can contribute towards a better lifestyle would be to incorporate some sort of exercise regiment into the daily or weekly schedule. Although a lot of people give excuses about not having the time for such activities, small changes can be made, such as learning to take the stairs whenever possible as compared to the alternative of using the elevators or escalators.

People often avoid healthy food choices mainly because of the perception that these foods are normally very bland tasting and rather boring. However with some careful thought and efforts such perceptions can be changed for the better.

Changing It

Getting children to adapt to healthier food choices can often be a very stressful event, but if such choices were taught to be made from a very early age then the battle will not be an all consuming as imagined. Preparing the healthier food to look and taste better would be the first way to encourage its consumption.

Making conscious decision to reach for healthier options when the opportunity presents itself is a discipline that should be advocated as much as possible. For the more innovative food preparation style there are some who go a step further to actually package the healthier foods to look and feel similar to the unhealthy food choice, an example of which would be presenting celery and carrot sticks in the packaging used to present French fries.

There are also some that package carrot sticks in cigarette boxes and berries in candy packaging. All these are conscious efforts made to play on the mental and visual effects of the individual, in the hope of encouraging the healthier choice being made.

Making other changes gradually such as consuming brown rice and whole-wheat products instead of white products is also another option to look into when making food choices. Having a couple of days dedicated to no meat consumption a week is another good start to make, and this can eventually progress to at least four days a week without meat, but this should not be done in succession as meat consumption is important to the body's needs. Adding more grains and nuts to the diet plan is also another healthy choice to make.

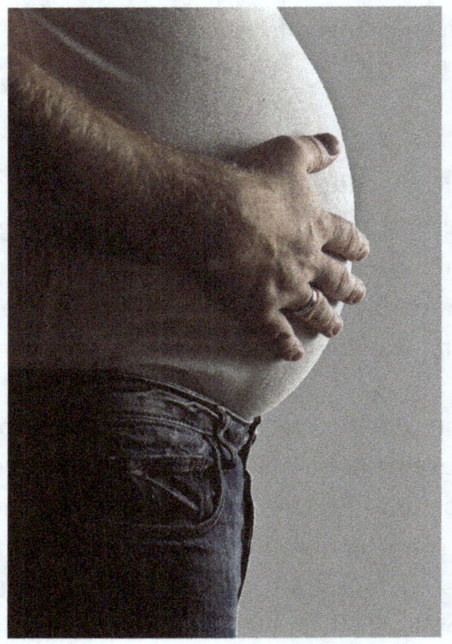

Chapter 7- Wellness, Healthy Lifestyle and Detoxification

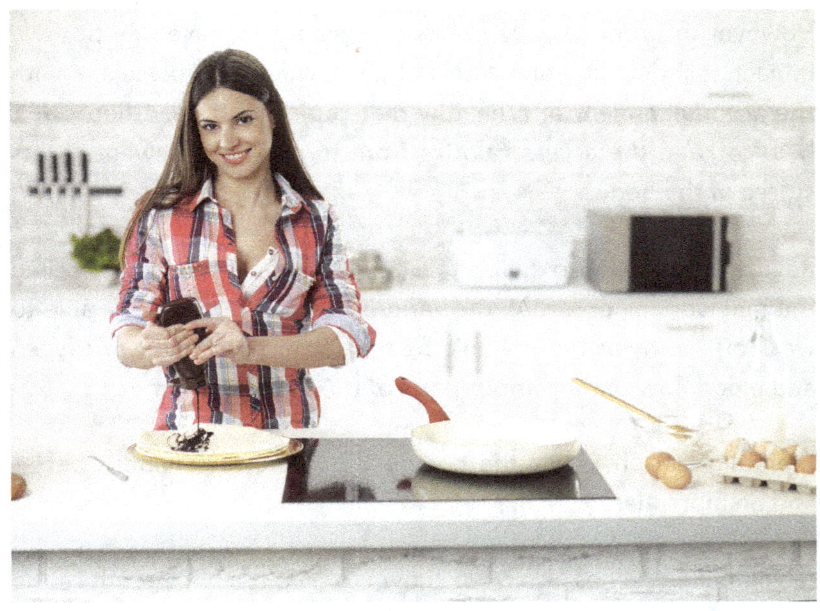

Exercise has long been advocated as an ideal way to stay healthy, next only to healthy food choices made for consumption. However for one reason or another, a lot of people do not seem to consider exercising an important part of the daily lifestyle schedule. This is an even more disastrous decision, when it is accompanied by poor diet habits.

Great Info

In the quest to stay healthy through regular exercise regiments, it may be prudent to take the time to understand just how an exercise regiment can contribute positively to the overall well being of an individual. The following are just some points on how exercise can contribute to a healthier lifestyle:

Regular exercise sessions can help to keep the body weight under control thus avoiding the possibility of gaining unnecessary weight and becoming overweight.

However in order for any exercise regiment to have any positive impact, it should be done with a regular schedule in place and with the accompaniment of a healthy diet choice, and only then can it help to keep the access calories from turning into unwanted fats stored in the body.

Regular exercise also helps to keep the body systems is prime optimal working order. All the various body systems will be able to work efficiently as there would be regular dispercement of oxygen and blood flow to the various parts of the body at all times.

Mentally and physically the body will be able to functions better and be more alert.

Regular exercise has also been known to help the body produce the necessary chemical make-ups that keep a good balance within the system. This essential chemical balance can contribute positively to the avoidance of negativity in the body system, without which, symptoms such as depression and mood swings are very likely to occur.

Detox Your Waste Away

The body naturally has its own detoxifying ways of getting rid of any negative residues left within the body system at regular intervals. However with the current lifestyles in place it is often difficult for the body to make such detox exercises complete and effective. Therefore there is a need to find other outside ways and means to help the body through the detox sessions.

Detox

Originally meant to eradicate the body system of alcohol and drugs there are now detox programs to actually help to recreate the optimum body conditioning for compete and better health. Such programs are fast gaining popularity and if used according to instruction the resulting conditions can be very impressive indeed.

Using certain diets, herbs and other specifically designed methods these detox programs help to remove any environmental and dietary toxins from the body system. Some of the ideas behind the use of these detox programs may include minimizing the amount of chemicals ingested which can be done with the consumption of just organic foods.

Another detox exercise would be designed around choosing foods that provide optimum vitamins, nutrient and antioxidants that the body needs to launch the detoxification exercise. There is also the detox program that contains foods such as those high in fiber and water to help draw out and eliminate toxins by increasing the frequency of bowel movements and urination.

All these efforts are needed to ensure optimum health simply because most adults live a lifestyle that is not very healthy to start with, thus the need for such invasive programs to keep the healthy balance in check.

Most people, who advocate the use of detox programs on a fairly regulatory schedule, attest to the overall better health conditions. These may be evident in better and clearer skin conditions, more energy, regular bowel movements, better digestion, increased levels of concentration and generally any other positive improvements felt.

Chapter 8- Begin your Healthy Lifestyle Now!

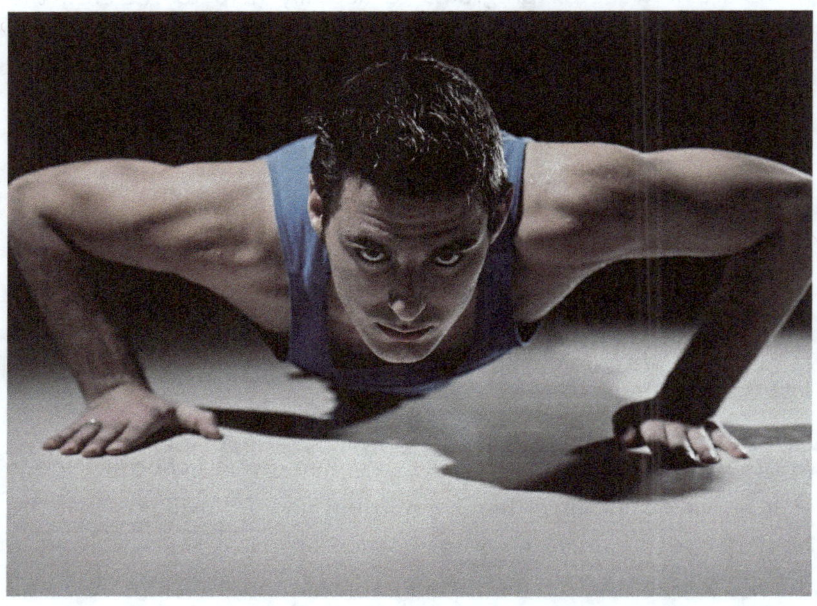

That's it… This is the entire 4-week program for building a lean, solid body. You now have all the tools you need to get started on an effective path to losing weight and getting in shape.

Between the Nutrition plan and this Workout plan, you can drop both pounds and body fat like crazy. If you stick to this plan and really bust butt for even a week, you can see noticeable differences in your body, muscle, and definition.

Depending on where you're starting from when you begin this program, your results will vary (they always do, no matter what). But here are some of the things you may experience after the 4 weeks are done – if you put in the work:

• A Flatter stomach (one a flat stomach, period!)

• More Muscle definition in your shoulders, arms, and legs

• A more defined jaw line

• Your clothes will fit better (be prepared to go shopping for new stuff)

• Confidence only a physically in-shape, attractive body can bring you (and the best part is that this will radiate out to other facets of your life as well)

These can all be yours! Follow the plan, commit to it in your mind and heart, and stay dedicated to it. Success is only hard work and dedication away.

Remember in the beginning I told you that you only need to do three things to lose weight successfully:

1) Restructure your diet

2) Workout in a way that burns fat while adding muscle

3) Build in a system of accountability

You now have a proven way to do all three of these. Follow the plan, stick to it, find your motivation, and hold yourself accountable.

You CAN do this!

No matter what, remember this:

A month from now, you'll wish you had started today.

Make the changes today that will get you closer to where you want to be tomorrow. That's all it takes. Small steps will get you to your destination, if only you keep taking them – daily, and with dedication.

Make today count!

About the Author

Wellness and restore you balance in and for life. This is what Helen Williams believes in order for you to enjoy and get more of life. Helen Williams is dedicated to educate and inspire all to bring back the zest in life through healthy lifestyle diet.

Helen Williams is a certified nutritionist and wellness coach. She also studied holistic Nutrition, Herbal and Natural Remedies, and Aroma Therapy.